21-DAY SUGAR

DETOX

Step-by-Step Guide to Quit Sugar the Smart Way

Sarah Green

1

Just to say "thank you" for buying this book, I'd like to give you a gift *absolutely free*

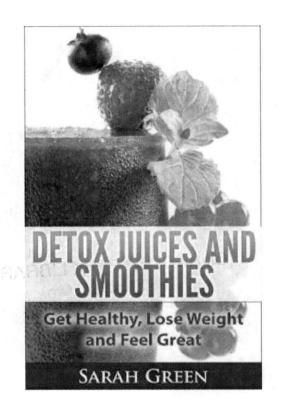

Get 5 Detox Juice and Smoothie Recipes from my best-selling book!

To claim your copy, simply go to:
www.alvobooks.com/sugardetox

Contents

Introduction

You've probably toyed with the idea of quitting sugar.

You've thought a lot about it.

You know you *should* do it.

But, at the end of the day, you feel overwhelmed, powerless, and don't know how to successfully tackle this life change.

I know what it feels like to suffer the health effects of sugar. When I was in my 20s, (which wasn't *that* long ago) I was totally addicted to candy, especially chocolate bars. Consuming large amounts of sugar was taking a toll on my body, and I didn't even realize it until I started feeling lethargic 24/7, my body turned from hourglass to pear, I had thrush all the time, and acne became a constant pain.

That's when I realized I needed to take control of my health. Within just a few weeks of cutting refined table sugar out of my diet, I felt vibrant and full of energy, and the acne and thrush were history. Better yet, I realized that my chances of contracting many serious and life-threatening diseases had been dramatically reduced.

I've changed my life and now I want to help you do the same.

Are you ready?

Ok, let's begin – say goodbye to sugar!

I know one of the reasons it took me so long to quit sugar was because it all seemed so overwhelming. I mean, I didn't have a clue how to start!

That's why I've developed this 21-Day Plan – all the information you need has been broken down so you can learn a little each day, plus there's a delicious juice, smoothie, or dessert recipe to enjoy. All the recipes have also been adapted for Paleo, gluten-free, and vegan diets, so everyone can enjoy them! This makes quitting sugar an absolute breeze because you just have to take a little step each day and, before you know it, you'll have achieved your goal.

Of course, if you're the type of person who likes to devour all the background info first and then get started, you can also choose to read the whole book in one go and then plan your sugar detox. Either way, you have all the information you need to kick that sugar habit!

Here's how it'll work:

In the first week we'll concentrate on learning about how refined sugar impacts our health, and we'll come to grips with the different types of sweeteners, the glycemic index, and sugar addiction.

In week two we'll get down and dirty with lots of practical tips on getting sugar out of your life for good. Plus there's really exciting information on foods that can actually help you quit sugar – you'll love it!

In the last week of the plan, we'll share even more valuable knowledge on how to live sugar-free, including how to eat out, how to replace sugar in your favorite recipes, and much more!

All the recipes in this book are for sugar-free sweet treats and delicious juices and smoothies that will accelerate your sugar detox. I wasn't going to disappoint you with a heap of salad recipes, because I know you're going to need something to satisfy your sweet tooth, especially at the start.

If you really want to boost your sugar detox results, you'll need to make sure your everyday diet is healthy. The key is to eat whole foods, as natural as possible. Let's put it this way; if you don't know what tree, plant, or animal a food has come from, give it a miss! You should aim to eat:

1. Fresh fruits and veggies
2. Lean meats, poultry, fish, and seafood
3. Free-range eggs
4. Natural nuts and seeds
5. Healthier grains like brown rice, quinoa, and oats
6. Healthy oils like extra-virgin olive oil, avocado oil, and coconut oil
7. Beans and legumes
8. Whole grain breads and pasta
9. Moderate amount of soy products like tofu, tempeh, and tamari
10. Moderate amount of dairy products like yogurt, cheese, and milk
11. Almond milk, soy milk, or any other non-dairy milk which is completely free from sweeteners of any type

12. Coconut milk, cream, and oil

Of course, exactly which items you eat from the above list will depend on other dietary constraints; I'm not suggesting you eat all of these foods, but I am saying that you should avoid foods that aren't on this list.

For example, I know that many of you follow the Paleo diet, so you'll obviously stick to your diet plan, which is great.

Other people are vegan, or gluten-intolerant, or lactose-intolerant, so you'll need to eat accordingly. Still others will be focused on losing weight, so you'll need to limit your intake of fattier foods like the oils and nuts.

The key is to maintain a diet based on whole foods and avoid anything processed. As we move through the book and talk in more depth about how the glycemic index works, along with other related vital information, you'll understand why.

I would also suggest that you avoid alcohol while on this 21-Day Sugar Detox. It's vital to stay hydrated while detoxing and you'll probably also experience some mild headaches or other sugar withdrawal symptoms, so why exacerbate this by drinking? It's also worth remembering that alcohol messes with your blood sugar levels. If you do choose to drink, however, there are some tips for making better choices on Day 20.

Of course, another vital consideration is how often you eat. Avoid skipping meals or going for prolonged periods without eating anything. This includes breakfast – even if you're busy and get up really early, at least grab a piece or fruit or some whole wheat crackers as you head out the door. Not eating makes you vulnerable and more likely to crave sugar. Aim to eat small meals often and make sure you have a healthy snack mid-morning and mid-afternoon.

OK, ready to get started?

Remember that those of you with health conditions (including diabetes and pre-diabetes) will need to plan your diet together with your health care practitioner.

Preparation

Set a Solid Foundation

Congratulations! You're about to start your 21-day sugar detox!

Choose Your Start Date Wisely
Before you embark on this 21-day sugar detox plan, check that today really is the best day to start. Now I'm not suggesting you needlessly postpone it, but unless you have an iron will, I'm going to suggest that you don't try and get started on Christmas Day, nor on your sister's wedding. Give yourself a head start by starting on a normal day, such as any old week day. As you continue on your sugar-free journey, you'll have the resources to deal with special occasions and tempting situations, but do yourself a favor and make it easy to get started.

OK, ready to move forward?

Make a Commitment
The first step in making any life change has got to be to make a committed decision. We all know what it's like to intend to do something, or know we should, but real change comes from making a firm decision and sticking to it. Making an open-ended commitment is also a recipe for disaster, which is why saying that you'll never eat sugar ever again probably won't work. Instead, make a commitment to 21 days sugar-free. This tangible amount of time is manageable, and knowing this will help you through any rough patches.

Mindset

Sometimes people can think "mindset" is some kind of new age or airy-fairy word, but it really just means your attitude. Do you have a positive attitude going into your sugar detox? Or do you think that you're going to fail? Are you concentrating on how it'll change your life for the better? Or are you telling yourself you're too weak to succeed?

What it boils down to is creating a positive, strong outlook and believing in yourself. Let's face it – a positive mindset or attitude will give you the best possible start and ensure your success in quitting sugar. If you're into affirmations, by all means, go ahead and use them. A more general strategy, though, is simply to be mindful of what you're saying to yourself. For example, if I catch myself saying something like, "this is too hard!" I simply flip the negative into a positive and tell myself, "I can do this!" Or if I'm out and I think, "there's sugar in everything! I can't find anything to eat!" I could change it to, "it's easy to find healthy sugar-free snacks".

Even if you're not a huge believer in mindset, I'm going to encourage you to have a go – I think you'll be amazed at the results!

Set Clear Boundaries

This book is predominantly intended for people who want to remove refined table sugar from their diet. For this reason, the recipes contain absolutely no cane sugar derivatives and no refined sugars. In addition, due to the health implications which we'll discuss later on, there are no artificial sweeteners. Instead, the recipes in this book use delicious natural fruits, dried fruits, raw honey, maple syrup, and stevia.

However, everyone's journey is different and you'll need to make decisions about what's right for you. The important thing is that you make these decisions beforehand, rather than when you have a dangerously tempting dessert in front of you. I invite you to set clear boundaries right now about what you will and won't consume.

Remember that those of you with health conditions (including diabetes and pre-diabetes) will need to make your plan together with your health care practitioner.

Day 1

Arm Yourself with the Facts

The best defense against sugar is the cold, hard knowledge of what it does to your body. It's a bit scary, but facing the facts makes it incredibly easy to say "no" to sugar.

Now I know some of you like things short and sweet, so here's the summary:

Consuming refined sugar is linked to:

1. Obesity
2. Diabetes
3. Heart Disease
4. Cancer
5. Chronic fatigue
6. Alzheimer's
7. Headaches
8. Tooth decay
9. Mood swings, anxiety, and irritability
10. Blurred vision
11. Dizziness
12. Cold sweats
13. Tremors
14. Drowsiness and/or insomnia
15. Candida
16. Acne

17. Infertility

18. Hypertension

19. …And the list goes on

If you're already sufficiently afraid, feel free to skip to today's tasty muffin recipe.

For those of you who love to get into the nitty-gritty, let's take a better look at some of the scientific research on the "lethal gifts" of refined sugar.

Diabetes

I wish I was wrong, but more than one in every three American adults is pre-diabetic.[1] This means that while they haven't developed type 2 diabetes yet, their blood glucose levels are abnormally high.

Here are some alarming facts from the National Diabetes Fact Sheet published by the National Center for Chronic Disease Prevention and Health Promotion:[2]

---

[1] "National Diabetes Factsheet", National Center for Chronic Disease Prevention and Health Promotion (2011), http://www.cdc.gov/diabetes/pubs/pdf/ndfs_2011.pdf (accessed January 10, 2014).

[2] "National Diabetes Factsheet", National Center for Chronic Disease Prevention and Health Promotion (2011), http://www.cdc.gov/diabetes/pubs/pdf/ndfs_2011.pdf (accessed January 10, 2014).

1. 25.8 million Americans are affected by diabetes, of which 7 million are undiagnosed.

2. The leading cause of heart disease, stroke, new cases of blindness, kidney failure, and non-traumatic lower-limb amputations is none other than diabetes.

3. Diabetes is the seventh leading cause of death in the US.

Sometimes when a condition like diabetes becomes widespread, it can almost be considered "normal". However, I'm sure you'll agree that there's nothing normal about suffering or dying from a preventable disease.

Obesity

More than two out of every three adults in the United States are overweight or obese.[3] Obviously, increased sugar consumption is one of the key causes of obesity.[4] Sugar contributes to weight gain not only because it is converted to fat, but also because it stimulates signals in the brain that make us believe we're hungry.[5]

---

[3] "Overweight and Obesity Statistics", Weight-control Information Network, http://www.win.niddk.nih.gov/publications/PDFs/stat904z.pdf (accessed January 10, 2014).

[4] "Obesity and Overweight", World Health Organization (2003), accessed January 10, 2014, http://www.who.int/dietphysicalactivity/media/en/gsfs_obesity.pdf

[5] Jeffrey Norris, "Sugar Is a Poison, Says UCSF Obesity Expert", UCSF (2009), https://www.ucsf.edu/news/2009/06/8187/obesity-and-metabolic-syndrome-driven-fructose-sugar-diet (accessed January 10, 2014).

Heart Disease

Did you know that a 20 oz. Coke has about fifteen teaspoons of sugar, while it's recommended that an adult man should consume no more than nine teaspoons, and an adult woman no more than six teaspoons, of added sugar per day?[6]

So, is the sugar in these sodas really *that* bad?

One recent study has revealed shocking facts. 40,000 men were examined for two decades and it was found that those who gulped a sugary beverage every day had a 20% higher risk of coronary heart disease than those who rarely consumed sugary drinks.[7]

Alzheimer's Disease

Alzheimer's disease is the most common and lethal form of dementia – and currently there is no cure for it. US researchers have found a link between Alzheimer's and high blood sugar – regardless of whether the person is diabetic or not.[8]

---

[6] "Added Sugars", American heart Association, http://www.heart.org/HEARTORG/GettingHealthy/NutritionCenter/Healthy DietGoals/Added-Sugars_UCM_305858_Article.jsp (accessed January 10, 2014).

[7] L de Koning, VS Malik, MD Kellogg, EB Rimm, WC Willett, and FB Hu, "Sweetened beverage consumption, incident coronary heart disease, and biomarkers of risk in men", Circulation. 2012;125:1735-41, S1. http://www.ncbi.nlm.nih.gov/pubmed/22412070 (accessed January 10, 2014).

[8] A Blue, "UA Research Suggests Link Between Elevated Blood Sugar, Alzheimer's Risk", UA News, http://uanews.org/story/ua-research-suggests-link-between-elevated-blood-sugar-alzheimer-s-risk (accessed January 10, 2014).

Cancer

Previously scientists could only speculate about the relationship between sugar and cancer. However, since certain sugar molecules were found in high numbers in cancer cells, this connection has now been confirmed. In co-operation with a research group from Singapore, scientists at the University of Copenhagen have revealed that certain sugar molecules actually cause the growth of cancer cells.[9]

Infertility

University of Utah biology professor Wayne Potts, along with Ph.D. student James Ruff, conducted a study on the effects of sugar consumption on mice.[10] When fed the equivalent amount of sugar consumed by 25% of Americans, the mice suffered from the effects of toxicity, including female mice dying at twice the normal rate, producing 25% less offspring compared to those that were fed a diet without added sugar, and male mice also suffered dramatically reduced fertility. Some people might argue that experiments on mice are not sufficient proof but professor Potts obviously sees the dangers as he has since reduced his – and his family's – sugar intake.

---

[9] "Specific sugar molecule causes growth of cancer cells", University of Copenhagen, http://news.ku.dk/all_news/2013/2013.9/specific-sugar-molecule-causes-growth-of-cancer-cells (accessed January 10, 2014).
[10] "Sugar is Toxic to Mice in 'Safe' Doses", The University of Utah News Center (2013), http://unews.utah.edu/news_releases/sugar-is-toxic-to-mice-in-safe-doses (accessed January 10, 2014).

Candida

Many women already instinctively know that there's a strong connection between sugar consumption and thrush, but there is also a lot of research to back this up. It has been proven that consuming refined sugars on a regular basis does indeed correlate with increased vaginal thrush.[11] The last thing anyone wants is a burning, itchy, inflamed vagina…

Acne

We all know it's true, and scientific research has also proven the link between sugar intake and acne.[12]

On a personal note, I suffered from severe acne for most of my 20s. I had absolutely no idea why at the time. Seeing as the dermatologist didn't ask about my diet, the connection didn't even occur to me. No, instead, his solution was to take a high dose contraceptive pill, when it turned out all I needed to do was cut my sugar consumption! It is absolutely insane to unnecessarily suffer from acne caused by excess sugar intake.

---

[11] BJ Horowitz, SW Edelstein and L Lippman, "Sugar chromatography studies in recurrent Candida vulvovaginitis",
http://www.ncbi.nlm.nih.gov/pubmed/6481700 (accessed January 29, 2014).
[12] RN Smith, NJ Mann, A Braue, H Mäkeläinen, and GA Varigos, "A low-glycemic-load diet improves symptoms in acne vulgaris patients: a randomized controlled trial", The American Journal of Clinical Nutrition (2007), http://ajcn.nutrition.org/content/86/1/107.full (accessed January 10, 2014).

Tooth Decay

According to a report by the American Dental Association, the average American drank more than 53 gallons of soda in 2000.[13] Americans drink more soda than any other beverage, including water!

Consuming large amounts of sugary drinks and foods makes your mouth acidic and it takes at least 20 minutes to return to its normal pH level. So, even if brush your teeth regularly but do not cut down on the intake of sugary foods and drinks, your teeth will be caught up in a constant battle against plaque and cavities.

Hypertension

Most people are aware of the link between salt and high blood pressure, but fail to realize that sugar is another culprit, and that this has been proven by scientific research. For example, a study conducted by the National Center for Biotechnology Information in 2010 confirmed that consuming sugary drinks increases blood pressure.[14] On a positive note, the study showed that the opposite was also true and that reducing soda intake lowers blood pressure.

---

[13] "Diet and tooth decay", American Dental Association (2002), http://www.ada.org/sections/scienceAndResearch/pdfs/patient_13.pdf (accessed January 10, 2014).
[14] L Chen et al, "Reducing Consumption of Sugar-Sweetened Beverages Is Associated with Reduced Blood Pressure: A Prospective Study among U.S. Adults", Circulation. June 8, 2010; 121(22), http://www.ncbi.nlm.nih.gov/pmc/articles/PMC2892032 (accessed January 10, 2014).

Anyone still craving sugar? I know I'm not.

Makes 12

Ingredients:
Oat bran – 1/2 cup
Coconut flour – 1 1/2 cups
Raw honey – 1/2 cup
Baking powder – 2 teaspoons
Nutmeg – 1 teaspoon
Eggs – 2
Almond milk – 1 cup
Coconut oil – 2 tablespoons
Vanilla extract – 1/2 teaspoon

<u>Special Diets:</u>
If you're on the Paleo diet or a gluten-free diet, use 1/2 cup almond flour to replace the oat bran.

If you're vegan, use 1/2 cup ground flax instead of the eggs, and add water as needed to form a sticky paste. You can replace the honey with maple syrup or any other sweetener of choice (see the substitute guide on day 18 for more ideas).

Directions:
1. Preheat your oven to 400°F (200°C) and coat your muffin tin with cooking spray.

2. Combine the oat bran, coconut flour, baking powder, and nutmeg in a bowl.

3. In a separate bowl, add the honey, milk, oil, egg whites, and vanilla extract into a bowl and whisk together well.

4. Pour the wet ingredients into the dry ingredients and combine. (Note: Some coconut flours are drier than others so, if the mixture ends up too dry, add a little water as needed).

5. Pour the mixture into the muffin tin, filling each cup about 3/4 full.

6. Bake for 15 minutes, or until a toothpick inserted in the center comes out clean.

Nutrition Facts per Serve:
Calories: 185
Carbs: 21 g
Fat: 3 g
Protein: 2.9 g
Sugars: 29.3 g

Day 2

Stay Hydrated

While we all know the importance of drinking eight glasses of water per day, staying hydrated is particularly important at the start of a sugar detox. This is because it'll prevent any withdrawal symptoms you experience – such as headaches – being exacerbated by dehydration. Drinking plenty of water also helps your body eliminate toxins, so you'll really give yourself the best possible start to your 21-Day Sugar Detox by doing this.

Of course, you can make water more exciting by adding a few fresh mint leaves, a couple of slices of lime, or berry ice cubes – I like to use blueberries and raspberries and just pop them in the tray with water and then freeze.

A great option in cooler months is to sip herbal tea. As well as keeping you hydrated, natural herbal teas can curb sugar cravings. Licorice root tea is an excellent choice because it curbs sugar cravings. Ginseng tea is another great option.

If you struggle to drink plain water, then vitamin water is a great alternative, especially for people who are used to drinking a lot of soda. Today's recipe is a great place to start…

Makes 8 cups

Ingredients:

Water – 8 cups

Lemon – 1, sliced thinly

Orange – 1, sliced thinly

Mint leaves – Handful, roughly chopped

Directions:

Place all the ingredients together in a jug and allow to sit overnight in the fridge.

Nutritional Facts per Serve:

Calories: 5

Carbs: 1.2 g

Fat: 0 g

Protein: 0.2 g

Sugars: 0.8 g

Day 3

Remember Why You're Doing This

On day one we went through the health problems associated with consuming refined sugar. Bet you swore off sugar on the spot, right? But I know it's tough at the start – especially in the first few days – and that sugar can start to seem tempting. That's why it's essential for you stay focused on why you're doing this.

Get out a small piece of cardboard or paper and pen because we're going to write. I know it might seem antiquated, but there's something about physically writing that makes things sink into your head better than just reading, and also better than typing.

Write the following:

I release sugar from my life and move into optimum health. I am energized, strong, and in perfect health. My skin is radiant and growing and I feel vital.

I suggest you carry this card with you in your purse and whenever you have a weak moment, take it out and read it; this will keep you focused on the positive changes you're making and help you stay focused. Don't worry if you feel a little silly at first because I did too. But it really helped, especially because I kept mine with my change in my purse, meaning I saw it every time I took money out...Very handy when you're tempted to buy candy!

Ingredients:

Papaya – 1 cup

Frozen blueberries – 1/2 cup

Almond milk – 1/2 cup

Directions:

Blend all the ingredients in your processor at high speed until smooth. This is one of my favorite breakfast smoothies!

Nutritional Facts per Serve:

Calories: 105

Carbs: 20.5 g

Fat: 0.2 g

Protein: 5.7 g

Sugars: 8.2 g

Day 4

Quitting Sugar

Exactly why is it so hard to quit sugar? Well, some researchers believe it can be as addictive as cocaine. A US study conducted in 2013 showed that rats exhibited the same level of addiction to Oreos as to cocaine. The researchers believe their results support the idea that high-sugar foods stimulate the brain in similar ways to drugs.[15]

But how does this work?

Sugar Addiction
The answer can be found in a study from Princeton University researchers in the March 2009 issue of the Journal of Addiction Medicine.[16] The study analyzed the animal model of sucrose addiction and found that it increases dopamine (a chemical involved in reward system feedback) in the brain. Sucrose also triggers the release of natural opioids which then enhance your mood. Based on these findings, the researchers concluded that

---

[15] "Student-faculty research suggests Oreos can be compared to drugs of abuse in lab rats", Connecticut College (2013), http://www.conncoll.edu/news/news-archive/2013/student-faculty-research-suggests-oreos-can-be-compared-to-drugs-of-abuse-in-lab-rats.htm (accessed January 10, 2014).

[16] Bartley Hoebel, Nicole Avena, Miriam Bocarsly, and Pedro Rada, "Sugar on the Brain: Study Shows Sugar Dependence in Rats", Jornal of Addiction Medicine Vol. 3 No. 1, (March 2009), http://www.princeton.edu/pr/news/02/q2/0620-hoebel.htm (accessed January 10, 2014).

when sucrose supply is cut, the dopamine levels drop and this probably leads to feelings of withdrawal.

You can beat sugar addiction, but you'll probably experience withdrawal. Although symptoms vary from person to person, it's common to experience fatigue, anxiety, mood swings, and intense cravings. The good news is that your cravings will end rather quickly – within three weeks of quitting sugar. This, my friends, is precisely why we're on a 21-day detox plan!

After that, you'll feel your energy levels increase and your moods stabilize. If you eat something with refined sugar, it will taste strangely synthetic and too sweet for your taste buds.

Emotional Sugar Fixes

We need to address another key issue at this point – the emotional connection with sugar. Many people find they use candy and other sweets to pick themselves up when they're feeling down. While it affects both sexes, women in particular are prone to this. How many times, for example, have you seen a friend go through a breakup, get fired, or suffer any other kind of emotional crisis, and the first thing we do to offer support is buy a tub of her favorite ice-cream or break out the cookie dough?

The first step is obviously recognizing the pattern. Then, you need to replace the use of sugar as a way of comforting yourself with a healthier habit. Getting out into the fresh air and going for a walk is a great option because exercise increases dopamine levels.

Calling a friend and chatting – without the sugar fix! – is another great option. Of course, if you're finding it tough, a short-term transition strategy is to use healthy recipes, like those in this book, to get a more natural sweet fix.

PMS

Many women experience distinctive cravings for sweets – especially chocolate – when they have PMS. I know I do. But I have a few strategies for dealing with these cravings. The first is magnesium supplements. It has been shown that taking 200mg of magnesium every day can alleviate a range of symptoms associated with PMS.[17] Personally, I've found magnesium supplements to alleviate candy cravings around my period. If I'm still craving sugar, though, I resort to eating 2-3 prunes. As these are high in iron, it's an excellent time to be eating them.

---

[17] AF Walker, MC De Souza, MF Vickers, S Abeyasekera, ML Collins, and LA Trinca, "Magnesium Supplementation Alleviates Premenstrual Symptoms of Fluid Retention", The American Journal of Clinical Nutrition (1998), http://www.ncbi.nlm.nih.gov/pubmed/9861593 (accessed January 10, 2014).

Stuffed Baked Apples
Serves 4

Ingredients:
Apples – 4 (I like to use red, but green are great as well)
Coconut butter – 2 tablespoons
Almond flour – 4 tablespoons
Ground cinnamon – pinch
Ground nutmeg – pinch
Pitted prunes – 1/2 cup, roughly chopped
Boiling water – 3/4 cup

Directions:
1. Preheat your oven to 375°F (190°C).

2. Remove the core from the apples.

3. Combine the coconut butter, almond flour, spices, and prunes in a bowl.

4. Line the apples up in a small baking dish. Stuff the apples with the almond and prune mixture.

5. Add the boiling water to the baking dish and bake for 30-40 minutes, or until tender (you can also make these apples in your slow cooker – cook on low for 3 hours).

Nutritional Facts per Serve:

Calories: 238

Carbs: 37 g

Fat: 8.7 g

Protein: 3.2 g

Sugar: 32 g

Day 5

Understanding the Glycemic Index

Instead of just analyzing foods according to the total amount of carbohydrates, the Glycemic Index (GI) is a more advanced means which looks at the actual impact of a certain food on our blood sugar level.

Foods are commonly categorized into three different classes: low GI (55 or less), medium GI (56—69), and high GI (above 70). Beans, whole grains, many fruits and veggies are some examples of low GI foods, dried fruits and bananas are some items with medium GI, and white bread and breakfast cereals are some foods with high GI.

Although the glycemic response varies from person to person and also depends on several other factors, generally speaking, eating low GI foods results in better blood glucose readings and so are ideal for your body.

According to Dr. David Jenkins,[18] foods with high GI have carbs that quickly break down during digestion and result in a rapid release of glucose into the bloodstream, while those with low GI

---

[18] DJ Jenkins, TM Wolever, RH Taylor, et al. "Glycemic index of foods: a physiological basis for carbohydrate exchange", American Journal of Clinical Nutrition 34.3 (1981), http://www.ncbi.nlm.nih.gov/pubmed/6259925 (accessed January 10, 2014).

break down slower and result in a gradual release of glucose into the bloodstream.

Good Carbohydrates

Good carbs are complex carbs that are composed of many chains of sugars joined together. Most good carbs are rich in fiber. Their complex structure and high ratio of fiber means the body takes long enough to break them down so that the bloodstream gets a steady supply of sugar. This enables the body to burn sugar for energy and keep energy levels and mood stable.

Some ideal sources of good carbs include fresh fruit and veggies, beans, and whole grains, which are rich in fiber, energy, vitamins, phytonutrients, and minerals.

Bad Carbohydrates

Simple carbs – aka bad carbs – are single or double-chained sugars, and usually end with an "ose" like fructose (from fruit), lactose (from dairy products), sucrose, and glucose. Simple carbs are usually found in low-fat foods, added for enhanced flavor. They hardly offer any vitamins, minerals, or phytochemicals. Owing to the simple structure and lack of fiber, your body quickly breaks them down and gets an instant boost in energy but then there is a sudden crash which results in unstable mood. Some examples of bad carbs include candy and soda.

What makes it slightly confusing is that not all simple carbs are "bad" carbs. For example, fruit contain simple carbs in the form of fructose, but this is mitigated by the fiber, minerals, vitamins, and enzymes they also contain. The same goes for dairy products. The danger is when these sugars are extracted from the whole food. So, the sugars in whole, natural grapes do not affect your body in the same way as processed, concentrated grape juice which is extracted and separated from the fiber.

Good Carbs Gone Bad

What makes it more confusing is the difference between refined and whole foods, such as whole grains. Whole grains have good carbs, but when refined, the nutrients and fiber are broken down which makes it easy for the body to digest, and hence makes it less nutritious. Likewise, corn has complex carbs and is good for the body, but commercial breakfast cereal and bread that have the same corn in refined form have bad (simple) carbs.

Tips to be on the Safe Side

Here are some simple tips to make sure you eat foods that have good carbs:

1. Avoid the lure of low-fat foods which often have added sugars
2. Avoid refined and processed foods
3. Eat carbs and protein together as this will lower glycemic response
4. Read labels and watch out for ingredients ending with "ose"

5. Go for smaller portions. Choose the smallest slice of bread and you'll eat about 20g less carbs per sandwich
6. Always choose whole wheat, brown or multi-grain
7. Eat fresh fruit, but in moderate quantities
8. Eat as many vegetables as you like (except starchy ones like potatoes and yams, which should be eaten in moderation)
9. Nuts, seeds, dairy products, beans, and pulses are also ideal low GI foods

Ingredients:
Chopped pineapple – 1 cup
Orange – 1/2
Natural yogurt – 1/2 cup
Ice – 1/2 cup
Vanilla extract – 1/2 teaspoon

<u>Special Diets:</u>
If you're on the Paleo diet, or are vegan or lactose intolerant, use 1/2 cup of coconut cream instead of yogurt.

Directions:
Combine all the ingredients in a blender and blend at high speed until smooth.

Nutritional Facts per Serve:
Calories: 176.5
Carbs: 32.3 g
Fat: 3.9 g
Protein: 5.7 g
Sugars: 21.5 g

Day 6

Types of Sweeteners

It's time for us to really understand all the sweeteners out there so we can make informed choices about what we want to consume. Let's take a quick look at some common sweeteners used in everyday foods.

Sugar Cane Sweeteners
Cane sugar is extracted from sugar cane mechanically, and results in several different products.

White Sugar
The first and most common type is refined white table sugar, also known as sucrose. It's a pure carb with energy content of 3.94 kcal per gram. It is one of the main culprits for all those health problems we discussed on day one.

Brown Sugar
The next most common type is brown sugar or raw sugar. It's partially refined and has a brownish color because of the presence of molasses. Although it's a common belief that brown sugar is better than white sugar, there is hardly any difference between the two. Brown sugar does have some calcium, potassium, iron, and magnesium, but only in extremely small amounts, so it hardly offers any health benefits. If you have to choose between white and brown sugar, brown wins by a whisker.

Demerara Sugar

Demerara sugar is a pale or golden yellow, partially refined sugar yielded during the first crystallization of cane juice into sugar crystals. Brown sugar has the added molasses flavor, while demerara tastes more like caramel. Again, to say it's healthier than white sugar is splitting hairs.

Muscovado Sugar

This sugar does not go through any centrifuge processes and so it is considered unprocessed. The sugar cane extract is simply heated and evaporated, so it does retain more minerals than other forms of cane sugar. While better than its refined cousins, don't fall into the trap of thinking that it can be freely consumed – it should still be used sparingly.

Golden Syrup

Another sweetener made in the process of refining sugar cane is called golden syrup. It's a thick, amber-colored sugar syrup and is somewhat similar in appearance to honey. It's amazing that some people suggest that you should consume golden syrup, because when you look at its components, you see that it contains three sugars i.e. sucrose (44%), fructose (27%), and glucose (27%). It has negligible nutritional value.

Palm Sugar

Palm sugar (also called jaggery) is made from the sap extracted from palm trees. Once the sap is extracted, it is then boiled until it thickens. It is much less refined than many cane sugar products, however, it still needs to be used sparingly.

Grain-Derived Sweeteners

There are several common types of grain-derived sweeteners including corn syrup, rice malt syrup, and barley malt syrup.

Corn Syrup

Corn syrup is made from maize starch and is high in fructose. It's the most commonly used sweetener in sodas and fruit-flavored drinks. There have been numerous studies linking high-fructose corn syrup to the current high rates of diabetes and obesity.[19] In fact, one study found that countries which use high-fructose corn syrup have been found to have rates of diabetes which are 20% higher. On top of that, it's processed using mercury and/or caustic soda, which can have a whole load of other health effects. This is one sweetener that you really need to keep away from.

Rice Malt Syrup

While rice malt syrup hasn't been linked to the issues associated with corn syrup, it's important to remember that it is still a processed product. Just think of a grain of brown rice and imagine what it goes through to end up as a liquid sweetener!

---

[19] L Ridgeway, "High fructose corn syrup linked to diabetes", USC (2012), http://news.usc.edu/#!/article/44415/high-fructose-corn-syrup-linked-to-diabetes/ (accessed January 10, 2014).

Barley Malt Syrup

Barley malt syrup is a sweetener produced by cooking sprouted barley malt. It has a lower GI index than common sugar and is less sweet. Previously it was considered safe and beneficial to health, but its major constituent is maltose, which is not very good for the body.

Plant-Derived Sweeteners

There are several different types of plant-based sweeteners, including maple syrup, agave nectar, and stevia.

Maple Syrup

Maple syrup is made from the sap of any of the different types of maple trees. Once collected, the sap is boiled down. It's believed to have some antioxidant properties and contains minerals such as zinc and manganese, but is also rich in sucrose. Maple syrup is a good natural sweetener, when used sparingly.

Agave Nectar

Agave nectar is a sweetener produced from a succulent plant called agave. The plant is native to Mexico and surrounding countries. The nectar contains small amounts of potassium, calcium, and magnesium, however, it is not significant nutritionally. Agave nectar can have up to 90% concentrated fructose, so it's potent and needs to be treated with care.

Stevia

Stevia is probably one of the best sweeteners, since it's almost 300 times sweeter than sugar, but has no calories, 0 GI, and virtually no effect on blood sugar. This plant is native to South America and has been safely used by indigenous people for centuries.

When the Bush administration gave stevia the green light to be used in soda and other flavored drinks, the Centre for Science in the Public Interest issued a statement that condemned this act, and labeled stevia as "potentially harmful".[20] However, no scientific evidence has yet been presented to prove the claim. Despite controversy in the US, stevia has been approved by both the World Health Organization and European Union. The WHO recommends a daily amount of 4mg per KG of body weight. [21] This amount was found to have no impact at all on blood glucose levels, even in people with type 2 diabetes.

Artificial Sweeteners

Artificial sweeteners – including aspartame, sucralose (which is sold under the name Splenda in the US, and appears on EU labels as E955), neotame, acesulfame potassium, and saccharin – are your worst enemy. Now I know this can be confusing, because many people believe that refined sugar is the worst sweetener you could ever put in your body. Unfortunately, artificial sweeteners also bring with them a whole host of problems.

---

[20] "FDA Issues Midnight Go-ahead for Potentially Harmful Stevia Sweetener", Center for Science in the Public Interest(2008), http://cspinet.org/new/200812181.html (accessed January 10, 2014).
[21] "Joint FAO/WHO Expert Committee on Food Additives", (2008), http://www.who.int/foodsafety/chem/jecfa/summaries/summary69.pdf (accessed January 10, 2014).

For example, aspartame has been deemed safe for human consumption by more than 100 different regulatory agencies, but several severe side effects including toxicity, blindness, hearing issues, memory loss, and seizures have been reported to the FDA.[22]

Saccharin, sold under the name Sweet'N Low, is another artificial sweetener commonly used in drinks, jams, candies, baked goods, cookies, medicines, and toothpaste. Amongst other potential health risks, it was banned for many years due to cancer fears. The FDA now claims that it's safe, and the fact that it causes cancer in animals allegedly doesn't mean it causes cancer in humans.[23] However, it's still banned in several other countries including Canada. While each person needs to make their own decisions about their health, I personally believe that the evidence remains firmly stacked against saccharin.

Sugar Alcohols
Sugar alcohols are water soluble solids commonly used in commercial foods in place of table sugar. There is a wide variety of sugar alcohols, however, the most common ones that you may find in so-called sugar free candy are maltitol, xylitol, lactitol, isomalt, and sorbitol.

---

[22] "Reported Aspartame Toxicity Reactions", 2003, http://www.fda.gov/ohrms/dockets/dailys/03/jan03/012203/02p-0317_emc-000199.txt (accessed January 10, 2014).
[23] LZG Touyz, "Saccharin deemed 'not hazardous' in United States and abroad". NCBI (2010), http://www.ncbi.nlm.nih.gov/pmc/articles/PMC3185898/#b1-conc-18-213 (accessed January 10, 2014).

Sugar alcohols are not alcohol, so don't worry, they won't get you drunk. They are, however, not completely absorbed by the body, and have less impact on your blood sugar compared to table sugar. Since your body doesn't break them down and digest them completely, sugar alcohols can be linked to several issues, including fermentation in the intestines, gas, diarrhea, and bloating. Sugar alcohols can also cause weight gain and raise the blood sugar levels of people with Type I diabetes.[24]

Honey

Honey is a natural, readily-available sweetener. Yes, it does have fructose and glucose, but it also has many other compounds, including antioxidants. Of course, the exact composition of honey varies depending on the specific bees and flowers used.

There have been some amazing studies on honey, including one conducted by the Journal of Medicinal Food in 2004 which compared honey with sucrose (table sugar) and dextrose. It was found that honey not only boosted HDL (good cholesterol) and lowered LDL (bad cholesterol) in diabetic patients, but also improved blood lipids and had minimal effect on glucose levels compared to sucrose.[25]

---

[24] "Eat any Sugar Alcohol Lately?", Yale-New Haven Hospital, http://www.ynhh.org/about-us/sugar_alcohol.aspx (accessed January 10, 2014).

[25] NS Al-Waili, "Natural honey lowers plasma glucose, C-reactive protein, homocysteine, and blood lipids in healthy, diabetic, and hyperlipidemic subjects: comparison with dextrose and sucrose", NCBI (2004), http://www.ncbi.nlm.nih.gov/pubmed/15117561 (accessed January 10, 2014).

While I of course respect that vegans prefer to avoid honey for ethical reasons, raw honey is an excellent sweetener for those who do consume animal products. When buying honey, always look for raw, untreated honey and be especially careful to avoid blends which mix honey with sugar syrup.

I hope this section on sweeteners has helped equip you so that you can make informed choices. Personally, I favor fresh and dried fruits, raw honey, maple syrup, and stevia. However, each person is different. Whatever choices you make, be sure to consider the available research about potential health impacts.

Fudgy Honey and Pecan Squares
Makes 40 bite-sized snacks

Ingredients:
Low fat cream cheese – 1 cup
Raw cocoa powder – 1/2 cup
Raw honey – 1/2 cup
Vanilla extract – 1 teaspoon
Pecans – 1/2 cup, roughly chopped

Special Diets:
If you're on the Paleo diet or are vegan or lactose intolerant, use 3/4 cup almond butter and 1/4 cup water instead of the cream cheese.

If you're vegan, instead of the honey, use 1/2 cup ground dates mixed with a little water to form a paste.

Directions:
1. Beat the cream cheese, raw cocoa powder, honey, and vanilla in a small bowl until combined into a smooth paste.

2. Then stir in the chopped pecans.

3. Spoon into a plastic container lined with plastic wrap. Put the lid on and refrigerate for at least 4 hours.

4. Cut into squares and serve chilled.

Nutrition Facts per Serve:

Calories: 39.5

Carbs: 4.7 g

Fat: 2.3 g

Protein: 1 g

Sugars: 3.6 g

Day 7

This is one of the most common questions I get asked, so let's get to the bottom of it.

Yes, your body does need sugar to have readily available fuel for your muscles and brain. The body also turns sugar into glucose to facilitate some basic bodily functions such as respiration and digestion.

But does this justify eating foods packed with sugar?

Absolutely not, because sugar is found in almost everything we eat, including foods with natural sugars like fruit, carbohydrates like bread, as well as vegetables and many other foods. So our body gets more than enough sugar from foods that don't have added sweeteners.

Do you have any idea how much sugar we eat nowadays? A lot…

The same amount of sugar which a person ate over five days in 1822 is now guzzled by an American in less than seven hours.[26] *That's more than 17 times as much sugar!*

---

[26] S Guyenet, "By 2606, the US Diet will be 100 Percent Sugar" (2012), http://wholehealthsource.blogspot.com.br/2012/02/by-2606-us-diet-will-be-100-percent.html (accessed January 10, 2014).

Sugar consumption is so out of control in the US that neurobiologist and obesity researcher Stephan Guyenet claims that if we continue to increase consumption at this rate, our diet will eventually consist of 100% sugar![27] If we live that long, of course.

Since refined sugar does not have nutritional value, its increased intake has decreased our intake of essential micronutrients[28] and played a key role increasing body weight.[29]

We are in absolutely no danger of failing to get the small amount of sugar necessary for proper bodily functions, and get more than we need from natural whole foods. In short, there is no reason to eat refined sugar.

---

[27] Ibid.

[28] BP Marriott, L Olsho, L Hadden, and P Conner, "Intake of added sugars and selected nutrients in
the United States", *National Health and Nutrition Examination Survey* (NHANES) 2003–2006.

[29] Jeffrey Norris, "Sugar Is a Poison, Says UCSF Obesity Expert", UCSF (2009), https://www.ucsf.edu/news/2009/06/8187/obesity-and-metabolic-syndrome-driven-fructose-sugar-diet (accessed January 10, 2014).

Afternoon Pick-Me-Up
Makes enough for you and a friend

Ingredients:
Pear – 1
Grapes – 1 cup
Celery – 2 stalks
Banana – 1
Fresh spinach – 1 handful
Cucumber – 1/2
Lemon juice – 1 tablespoon
Ice – 1 cup

Directions:
Process all the ingredients in a high-powered blender until smooth and serve.

Nutrition Facts per Serve:
Calories: 123
Carbs: 34 g
Fat: 0.5 g
Protein: 2 g
Sugars: 12 g

Congratulations – you've just made it through your first week!

Now I know it probably wasn't completely smooth sailing, so I'm sure you'll be pleased to hear that the first week is usually the hardest – it was for me.

OK, one week down, two more to go…
I hope you're as excited as I am!

Day 8

Beware the Wolf in Sheep's Clothing

Soda...Yes, Even Diet!

Advertising campaigns from companies like Coca Cola would like us to believe that we need the "positive energy" in sugar, however, the truth is rather ugly. Yesterday we got to the bottom of the myth that we "need" refined sugar in our diet, and you should have already cut out regular soda on day one.

However, if you think diet soda is safe, consider the fact that people who drink diet soda actually end up consuming more calories.[30] Ironic, isn't it? Remember how we talked about the fact that artificial sweeteners stimulate your appetite? Well, that's why diet soda makes you pile on the pounds. Of course, there are also all the health problems associated with artificial sweeteners, which are major cause for concern in their own right.

Fruit Juice

While we're at it, we need to look at another hidden danger – juice.

---

[30] D Sara N. Bleich, Julia A. Wolfson, Seanna Vine, and Y. Claire Wang, "Diet-Beverage Consumption and Caloric Intake Among US Adults, Overall and by Body Weight", American Public Health Association (2013) http://ajph.aphapublications.org/doi/abs/10.2105/AJPH.2013.301556 (accessed January 10, 2014).

Let's be clear that not all juice is created equal. Of course, the healthiest option is to eat fresh, whole fruit. The next best thing is smoothies made right before you drink them, which contain all the fiber of the whole fruit. After that, the next best thing is fresh juices made right before serving, especially if they contain a mix of fruit and veg. All of these are fine as part of a balanced diet.

The culprit we're talking about here is processed fruit juice, the type you buy in cartons in the supermarket. This "juice" is often packed with hidden sugars, artificial sweeteners and additives, and can have significant impacts on your health.

Even though the word "juice" sounds healthy, we need to learn to distinguish good juices from bad ones. Basically, if you make it at home in your juicer or blender – or you see it being made in front of you – and it just consists of whole, natural produce, you're good to go. If you have no idea when it was made and it comes with preservatives and strange ingredients you can't identify, give it a miss.

Alternatives

People often ask me what they should drink instead of sugary drinks. My answer is simple: drink water. Yes, water. It may seem radical but your body needs 8 glasses of water each and every day, so give it what it needs!

This is a big change for many people, but one well worth making to ensure both your health and your family's health. If you're having a really hard time trying to wean your kids off soda, you could consider switching to fruit juice and then gradually diluting it with more and more water. After a few weeks they'll be drinking almost pure water with only a dash of juice (hint: using a strong-colored juice helps visually fool them) and then it'll be easy to get them onto 100% water.

Another great alternative is vitamin water, which we talked about on day two. Another great option is today's delicious lemonade recipe.

Ingredients:
Juice of 1/2 lemon
Tomato – 1
Watermelon – 1 1/2 cups

Directions:
Process all the ingredients in a blender and serve. In summer it's nice to add 1/2 ice to the mix as well.

Nutrition Facts per Serve:
Calories: 86
Carbs: 21.9 g
Fat: 0.5 g
Protein: 2.2 g
Sugars: 16.8 g

Day 9

Complete Clean Out

If you're like I was, you probably have some scary hidden sugar lurking in your kitchen, or maybe even in your bedside drawers, in your car glove box, or on your desk at work or, well, anywhere else you like to hide it!

It's really simple – if you get rid of it all, you'll never have to fight temptation in a weak moment.

Start with the obvious culprits like all the cookies, candy, and chocolate bars but then there are some foods lurking in your kitchen such as processed oatmeal, corn flakes and processed cereals, granola, salad dressing, ketchup, pasta sauce, barbecue sauce, along with most other processed sauces and condiments, some soy milk and nut milks, some yogurts, peanut butter, commercial breads, canned and preserved fruits and vegetables, and sports drinks that you might not even consider when trying to get rid of hidden refined sugar.

Until you get used to which brands are safe, you'll have to spend a little time reading labels. Of course, the easiest way to avoid this hassle is to buy whole foods – you don't have to read an apple to know what's in it!

To give you a special incentive to clean out, I've got a super easy and delicious berry ice-cream recipe for you today. Hint:

Put your ingredients in the freezer before you start clearing out the kitchen and then you'll be ready for your reward when you're done.

Berry Delicious Ice-Cream
Makes enough for 2 people

Ingredients:
Frozen berries – 1 cup
Frozen bananas – 2
Skim milk (or nut milk) – 1/4 cup

Directions:
Blend all the ingredients in your food processor at high speed until smooth. You should have a super smooth and creamy ice-cream. If it gets too liquid while processing, simply put it back in the freezer for 20 minutes before serving.

Nutritional Facts per Serve:
Calories: 153
Carbs: 36 g
Fat: 0.3 g
Protein: 3.1 g
Sugars: 18.6 g

Day 10

Eat More Fiber

Fiber is important for many reasons. In relation to sugar, fiber makes you feel full, promotes healthy bowel movements, and also stops your gut from absorbing too much carbohydrate. Eating more fiber also helps reduce sugar cravings, which is vital during this 21-Sugar Detox.

What does this mean in practice?

Use the Whole Fruit
Whole fruit is always better than juice. "Juice" made by blending whole fruit with water is better than juice extracted from the flesh using a juicer.

Speaking of fruits, it's wise to focus on fruits that have a higher percentage of fiber compared to fructose. For example, raspberries, blueberries, pears, and kiwi fruit all contain really healthy ratios of fiber to fructose. All fruits can be enjoyed in moderation, but it's worth being aware that some have more fiber and less natural sugar.

Incorporate High-Fiber Foods
A great source of fiber which leaves you feeling full can be found in pulses and legumes. Some great choices are garbanzo beans and kidney beans, along with any other lentils or beans.

Prunes, almonds and other nuts, whole grains, veggies (especially broccoli, carrots, and celery), and flax seeds are all excellent sources of fiber.

Drink Plenty of Water
When you eat a high-fiber diet, it's essential to drink enough water. This is because fiber absorbs water, so you need to have enough available for proper digestion.

Increase Fiber Gradually
Like any other changes to your diet, it's best to gradually increase the amount of fiber you eat. That way the change will be comfortable and you won't experience any digestive repercussions, if you get my drift!

Oaty Fruit and Nut Cookies
Makes around 24 cookies

Ingredients:
Rolled oats – 1 cup
Oat bran – 2 tablespoons
Whole wheat flour – 1 cup
Eggs – 2
Baking powder – 2 teaspoons
Vanilla extract – 1 teaspoon
Chopped walnuts – 1/2 cup
Chopped dates – 1/2 cup
Raisins – 1/2 cup
Coconut oil – 2 tablespoons
Water – 1/2 cup

<u>Special Diets:</u>

If you're on the Paleo diet or a gluten-free diet, use 1 cup almond flour, 1/2 cup tapioca starch and 1/2 cup of coconut flour to replace the oats, oat bran, and wheat. If you're not a fan of tapioca starch, you can substitute 1/2 cup finely ground flax.

If you're vegan, use 1/2 cup ground flax instead of the eggs, and add water as needed to form a sticky paste.

Directions:

1. Preheat your oven to 375°F (190°C) and line a baking sheet with parchment paper.

2. Blitz your oats in your food processor to make a fine flour.

3. Combine the dry ingredients in a bowl (oats, oat bran, flour, and baking powder).

4. Form a well in the middle and add the eggs, oil, and vanilla. Mix until combined.

5. Add around 1/2 cup water, or sufficient to form a thick batter (the exact amount will depend on the brands of your dry ingredients etc.).

6. Lastly, add the raisins, chopped walnuts, and chopped dates and mix through.

7. Place spoonfuls of the mixture onto your lined baking sheet, then bake for 15-20 minutes, or until golden brown.

8. Enjoy your sugar-free, highly fibrous, and extremely delicious cookies!

Nutrition Facts per Serve:
Calories: 121
Carbs: 18 g
Fat: 6.3 g
Protein: 2 g
Sugars: 30.5 g

Day 11

Counter Attack by Getting Active

One of the best ways of beating sugar cravings and withdrawal is by getting active. This is because exercise stimulates a lot of the same feel-good chemicals in your brain that sugar does, such as dopamine. Working out also stimulates serotonin and the release of endorphins, which brings about the same great feeling some people seek through candy or other sweetened foods, and increases oxygenation.

So, going for a walk, hitting the gym, going for a swim, going to a yoga or Pilates class, or any other kind of exercise is a great way to get your mind off sugar cravings. Even a short stroll around the block can really help – you'll be surprised! Not only will your sugar cravings be history, but you'll also shed some weight and improve your general health and fitness.

Ingredients:
Celery – 2 stalks
Cilantro – 1 handful
Cucumber – 1
Green apple – 1

Directions:
Process all the ingredients in a juicer and enjoy.

Nutrition Facts per Serve:
Calories: 88
Carbs: 24.5 g
Fat: 0.7 g
Protein: 0.3 g
Sugars: 17.6 g

Day 12

Unite and Conquer

By now you're probably pretty freaked out about the health problems related to sugar and are not just thinking about your own health, but also that of your friends and family.

Family

If you have kids, you'll naturally be worried about their health and future. While quitting sugar by yourself still provides a good role model, the best thing is to unite as a family and do it together. Talk to your kids. Even if they're young, you can still explain the changes you're making, even to a 3 or 4 year old. Put it in their language; ask them if they want to learn how to get big and strong, run fast, and jump real high. Tell them some foods make people sick and some make them strong, and ask whether they want to be sick or strong. Say that you're all learning together as a family and make sure you include them in the learning experience. Of course, you might also have to be prepared to weather any short-term tantrums for the long-term health of the whole family.

If you have teenagers, you'll have to take a different approach – trying to convince them of anything will probably just have the opposite effect! Instead, set a good example by your actions, because we all know actions speak louder than words. Simply having healthier food choices available in your home will have a significant impact on what they eat every day. Of course, a really effective way of getting them interested is to casually let them know how diet affects things like acne – this is something every teenager would love to get rid of!

Friends

If you live with friends or roommates, let them know what you're doing and why, and if they're interested, get them to join you. Or if you have close work colleagues, see if any of them want to quit sugar together. Having a good support network makes it much easier to make this life changing move. It also makes it more fun because you can share your wins and improved health with others, as well as share recipes.

Avoid Preaching

A word of warning: mention that you're quitting sugar to your friends and loved ones but don't become an evangelist and try and convert them. Everyone is at different stages on their life journey. In fact, the best thing you can do is make positive changes in yourself, and model a healthy lifestyle. Everyone wants to look and feel great, and you can be sure that people will notice and start asking what you're doing.

Moist Apple Muffins
Makes 12

Ingredients:

Whole wheat flour – 2 cups

Baking powder – 2 teaspoons

Apples – 2 minced

Raw honey – 4 tablespoons

Skim milk (or soy or nut milk) – 3/4 cup

Eggs – 2

Coconut oil – 2 tablespoons

Ground cinnamon – 1 teaspoon

Ground nutmeg – Pinch

Vegetable cooking spray

<u>Special Diets:</u>

If you're on the Paleo diet or a gluten-free diet, use 1 1/2 cups almond flour and 1/2 cup tapioca starch to replace the wheat flour. Another alternative is 1 1/2 cups coconut flour and a mashed banana.

If you're vegan, use 1/2 cup ground flax instead of the eggs, and add water as needed to form a sticky paste. You can replace the honey with maple syrup or any other sweetener of choice (see the substitute guide on day 18 for more ideas).

Directions:

1. Preheat your oven to 360°F (180°C) and coat your muffin tin with cooking spray.

2. Combine the flour, baking powder, and spices in a bowl.

3. In a separate bowl, beat the honey, milk, oil, and eggs until combined (if your honey is hard, microwave for 10 seconds to loosen it up).

4. Pour the wet ingredients into the dry ingredients and combine.

5. Add the minced apple to the muffin batter and mix through.

6. Pour the mixture into the muffin tin, filling each cup about 3/4 full.

7. Bake for around 15-20 minutes, or until a toothpick inserted in the center comes out clean.

Nutrition Facts per Serve:
Calories: 132
Carbs: 17 g
Fat: 3 g
Protein: 3 g
Sugars: 16.3 g

Day 13

Distract Yourself

As I mentioned earlier, quitting sugar is a tough row to hoe and you'll probably experience some cravings. Sometimes the safest bet is to divert your attention. If you crave a candy bar or dessert, pick up a magazine or book, watch a movie, or call a friend.

The easiest way to stop thinking about candy is to start thinking about something else.

Let me tell you from experience – trying *not* to think about sugar doesn't work. This is because your brain doesn't hear the negative word "don't", and so it naturally brings up thoughts of every sugar-filled treat you've ever seen. You know how when you tell a young kid "don't run" or "don't yell" they do exactly what you don't want them to do? Well, us big kids are the same. Instead, start focusing on positive activities and other things you enjoy to take your mind off sugar.

If you love craft, start an exciting new project. If you love your dogs, spend time taking them for extra-long walks. Whatever you're into, take this opportunity to immerse yourself in doing what you love.

Ingredients:
Strawberries – 1 cup
Banana – 1
Natural yogurt – 1/2 cup
Ice – 1/2 cup

<u>Special Diets:</u>
If you don't eat dairy, use coconut cream instead of yogurt – it's delicious!

Directions:
Blend all the ingredients in your processor at high speed until smooth.

Nutritional Facts per Serve:
Calories: 190
Carbs: 47.2 g
Fat: 0.9 g
Protein: 8.7 g
Sugars: 21.3 g

Day 14

10 Foods That Help You Quit Sugar

I bet you're super excited to hear that there are foods that actually help ease sugar cravings and make the process of quitting sugar easier! Wow. Now I've already been sneaking some of these foods into your daily recipes, but here's a list of ten great ingredients to include in your diet.

1. *Cinnamon*: Thanks to the high amount of hydroxychalcone in cinnamon, it helps enhance the effects of insulin, which satisfies your sugar cravings to a great extent. Research has found another amazing fact about cinnamon – it actually has positive effects on blood glucose levels! [31]

2. *Tomatoes*: Low serotonin levels are one of the biggest reasons behind sugar cravings, which is where tomatoes come in handy, as they are naturally rich in serotonin. Tomatoes also have a high concentration of chromium – another mineral that minimizes food cravings and moderates blood sugar.

3. *Broccoli*: Just like tomatoes, broccoli is also rich in chromium – essential for proper insulin function and moderating your blood sugar.

---

[31] B Mang, M Wolters, B Schmitt, K Kelb, R Lichtinghagen, DO Stichtenoth, and A Hahn,
"Effects of Cinnamon Extract on Plasma Glucose, HbA, and Serum Lipids in Diabetes Mellitus Type 2", NCBI (2006),
http://www.ncbi.nlm.nih.gov/pubmed/16634838 (accessed January 10, 2014).

4. *Spinach*: Ever saw Popeye the sailor eat spinach and recharge his superhuman strength? Well, I'm sorry to tell you that you might not become a superhuman by eating this leafy green, but you can expect controlled blood glucose levels because of the rich amounts of magnesium found in spinach.

5. *Spirulina*: Spirulina is a type of bacteria (specifically a cyanocabteria, not an algae as commonly believed). Since it's high in tryptophan, research has found that it helps control blood sugar levels.[32] You can buy it from health food stores and drug stores either as a supplement, a powder, or in flakes. I usually buy it as a powder because it's easy to stir into smoothies, juices, and even yogurt. It turns food a scary green color, but is pretty mild in taste if you just use half a teaspoon or so.

6. *Pineapple*: This is of my favorite fruits…It's rich in manganese and fiber, and also has several essential vitamins and nutrients. The manganese and fiber in pineapple improve cholesterol levels and maintain blood sugar levels.

7. *Sesame seeds*: Sesame seeds are an ideal source of zinc and several other minerals which can play a key role in stopping blood sugar spikes. Sprinkle toasted sesame seeds over salads

---

[32] P Parikh, U Mani U, and U Iyer, "Role of Spirulina in the Control of Glycemia and Lipidemia in Type 2 Diabetes Mellitus", NCBI (2001), http://www.ncbi.nlm.nih.gov/pubmed/12639401 (accessed January 10, 2014).

and stir fries and add tahini (sesame paste) into smoothies, cookies, and desserts.

8. *Avocados*: As a healthy source of monounsaturated fat, avocados improve insulin sensitivity and prevent sugar cravings.

9. *Licorice*: Licorice is a versatile herb used in both cooking and herbal medicines. Note that we're talking about the plant, not the sticky black candy! Licorice root has a natural sweetness that stops your sugar cravings without raising blood sugar levels and makes an excellent herbal tea.

10. *Ginseng*: This Asian herb is conventionally used to boost energy levels for people suffering from chronic ailments. Being a central nervous system stimulant, it can not only lower your blood sugar level but also be useful in overcoming sugar addiction.

Nutty Banana Spinach Smoothie
Makes enough for you and a friend

Ingredients:
Baby spinach – 1 1/2 cups
Almond milk – 1 1/2 cups
Banana – 2 medium
Tahini (sesame paste) – 2 teaspoons
Spirulina – 1 teaspoon

Directions:
Blend all the ingredients in your food processor at high speed until smooth.

Nutritional Facts per Serve:
Calories: 178
Carbs: 28.5 g
Fat: 21.1 g
Protein: 3.3 g
Sugars: 14.4 g

Wow – you've already made it through two whole weeks!
Congratulations!

Give yourself a pat on the back - only one more week to go to get refined sugar out of your system for good.

Day 15

12 Simple Tips on How to Shop

You've cleaned out your kitchen, but now you have to make sure you keep your home stocked with healthy food. Let's see how:

1. You know how people always say you should never go shopping on an empty stomach? Well, it's true! Don't do it! Seriously, going to the supermarket when you're starving is just plain asking for trouble. Instead, go right after you've had a nice filling meal.

2. Before you head to the grocery store, write out your menu for the week and make a shopping list of everything you actually need. Creating a shopping list at home and not including any unhealthy, sugar-rich foods will make ignoring dangerous items easier when you're in the supermarket.

3. Better yet, avoid temptation all together and shop online. Not only will you guard against impulse buys, you'll also bypass the queues!

4. Buy whole foods – if you don't know what plant or animal the product comes from – don't buy it.

5. When in the bakery, always go for whole wheat and multigrain breads. Pitta breads, sourdough, rye bread, and

chapattis are also pretty good options. Don't forget that you still need to read the labels as there are heaps of whole wheat options that look healthy at first glance – until you read the ingredients and discover what's hidden in them...

6. A good tip is to start in the fruit and veggie section and fill most of your cart before even venturing into the other aisles – this will ensure you're maximizing the amount of healthy food you buy.

7. Don't waste your money on special diabetic or sugar-free products such as diabetic candy or chocolate because they're usually not worth the extra cash and are full of dangerous artificial sweeteners.

8. I suggest that you refrain from drinking on this 21-Day Sugar Detox but, if you do drink alcohol, you need to be careful of the choices you make. Avoid premixed drinks and go for dry red wine or spirits. Check out the alcohol tips on day 20 for more ideas.

9. When buying packed items, reading labels is very important because almost all processed foods have high fructose, corn syrup, or other types of refined sugar. We'll talk about reading labels in detail tomorrow, but a good guideline is that the fewer the ingredients, the better, and the ingredients should be recognizable whole foods rather than words you need a chemistry degree to understand.

Pay special attention to:

Granola, ketchup, mustard, sauces, salsa, mayonnaise, salad dressing, energy bars, yogurt, processed meat, margarine, peanut butter, soy and nut milks, canned and dried soups, bouillon cubes and stock, canned fruit and veg, and anything allegedly sugar-free (which is probably loaded with artificial sweeteners).

10. If you have a hectic lifestyle and struggle to find time to cook healthy meals, simplify your life by buying frozen spinach and peas, and pre-washed salad greens. These items are nutritious and make preparing meals much faster. Stock up on sugar-free canned beans and canned tomatoes as these are other healthy ingredients that make cooking a breeze.

11. Shopping at farmer's markets means you'll only go home with fresh, whole foods, and completely avoid all the processed foods lurking in supermarkets – give it a try.

12. Another suggestion is to subscribe to a fruit and vegetable delivery service and get a box of healthy produce delivered to your door every week. We're all busy and juggling a thousand things, so why not make it easy to have healthy options on hand?

Ingredients:
Green apple – 1
Celery – 4 stalks
Cucumber – 1
Kale – 5 leaves
Ginger – 1/2 thumb

Directions:
Simply process the ingredients in a juicer and serve!

Nutrition Facts per Serve:
Calories: 103
Carbs: 24 g
Fat: 0.1 g
Protein: 3.1 g
Sugars: 19 g

Day 16

Know Thy Enemy: Names of Sweeteners

Unfortunately, identifying sweeteners on a label can be tough because food manufacturers deliberately use a host of other words to try and make it seem like their products don't contain as much sugar and as many sweeteners as they really do. Here's a list of words to watch out for:

Amasake
Cane crystals
Cane sugar
Caramel
Caramelized foods
Carbitol
Concentrated fruit juice
Corn sweetener
Corn syrup
Crystalline fructose
Dextrin
Dextrose
Diglycerides
Disaccharides
D-tagalose
Evaporated cane juice
Florida crystals
Fruit juice concentrates
Fructooligosaccharides

Fructose

Galactose

Glucitol

Glucoamine

Gluconolactone

Glycerides

Glycerine

Hexitol

High-fructose corn syrup

Inversol

Invert sugar

Inverted sugar syrup

Isomalt

Karo syrups

Lactose

Levulose

Malitol

Malt syrup

Malted barley

Maltodextrins

Maltodextrose

Maltose

Malts

Mannitol

Mannose

Microcrystalline cellulose

Molasses

Monoglycerides

Monosaccarides

Nectars

Pentose

Polydextrose

Polyglycerides

Powdered sugar

Raw sugar

Ribose rice syrup

Rice malt

Rice syrup solids

Saccharides

Sorbitol

Sucanat

Sucrose

Trisaccharides

Xylitol

Zylose

No wonder we're confused! To make it even worse, this list isn't even exhaustive – there are other names! The best guideline is to avoid products with ingredients that you don't understand. After all, even if they're not a form of processed sugar, these industrialized additives are unlikely to be good for you.

After that scary list of sugars, I thought we could do with a sweet treat that we can understand – fruit popsicles! These popsicles are naturally sweet because of the whole, nutritious fruit in them.

This recipe is best made with a popsicle mold and yields 12 small.

Ingredients:
Mango – 1 large and very ripe
Peaches – 4
Water – 1 1/2 cups

Directions:
1. Peel the mango and remove the seed. Blend in your food processor with the water.

2. Slice the peaches and distribute them evenly among the molds.

3. Pour the blended mango mixture over the peaches until the molds are almost full (remember they'll expand a little once frozen).

4. Remove any air bubbles by gently tapping the molds.

5. Freeze (this will take 4 – 6 hours).

Nutrition Facts per Serve:

Calories: 25

Carbs: 6 g

Fat: 0.1 g

Protein: 0.4 g

Sugars: 5.3 g

Day 17

Ever get confused by the weird info mentioned on the food labels? Let's make sure it doesn't happen from here on. Even though this book is on quitting sugar, it's still useful to understand food labels, so we'll cover all the general aspects as well as those related to sugar.

General Guidelines

Here are some simple guidelines to help you read and understand labels:

1. Items are listed in descending order, in other words, the main ingredients are at the top of the list. So if you find sugar, corn syrup, dextrose or other sweeteners near the top of the list, it's a clear signal of the high amount of added sugar.

2. Be aware that sugar can have many different names and that the labels on processed foods often try to trick consumers by using less obvious ones. Remember all those tricky names in yesterday's reference list? Beware…

3. Instead of just looking at the sugars, look at the ratio of sugar and total carbs because some nutritious foods such as fruit do contain some natural sugar.

89

4. Remember that high-fiber foods help maintain stable glucose levels in your body, so consider the amount of fiber as well.

Nutrition Facts

Serving Size 1 cup (228g)
Servings Per Container 2

Amount Per Serving

Calories 250	Calories from Fat 110

% Daily Value*

Total Fat 12g	18%
Saturated Fat 3g	15%
Trans Fat 1.5g	
Cholesterol 30mg	10%
Sodium 470mg	20%
Total Carbohydrate 31g	10%
Dietary Fiber 0g	0%
Sugars 5g	
Protein 5g	

Vitamin A	4%
Vitamin C	2%
Calcium	20%
Iron	4%

* Percent Daily Values are based on a 2,000 calorie diet. Your Daily Values may be higher or lower depending on your calorie needs:

	Calories:	2,000	2,500
Total Fat	Less than	65g	80g
Sat Fat	Less than	20g	25g
Cholesterol	Less than	300mg	300mg
Sodium	Less than	2,400mg	2,400mg
Total Carbohydrate		300g	375g
Dietary Fiber		25g	30g

Deciphering Food Labels

Let's crack the different items on a food label.

Serving size

This is a standardized measurement based on the amount people generally eat at a given meal. However, the amount you eat may be different, and the "standard" serving size may be incredibly small, especially for snack foods. It's good to understand this concept, because the nutrients are mentioned according to one standard serving. So if you eat more than the amount mentioned on the label, you're probably consuming more sugar and so forth than you realize.

Calories

Calories are how much energy you'll get from each serving, while calories from fat are how much of that energy is coming from fat alone.

Total Fat, Saturated Fat, and Trans Fat

Total fat gives you the total amount of fat (good fats like mono or polyunsaturated fats as well as bad fats like saturated and trans fats) per serving. Good fats lower blood cholesterol levels while bad fats increase it, along with the chances of heart disease and other health problems. Pay careful attention to what types of fat are in products.

Cholesterol

How much cholesterol the particular food has is mentioned here. It goes without saying that you should favor foods with low cholesterol.

Sodium

Sodium, or salt, should be consumed in moderation. Unfortunately, processed foods tend to be very high in sodium.

Total Carbohydrate

The total amount of all types of carbs including carbs from sugar, complex carbs, and those with fiber is listed here. Because carbs can affect your blood sugar, it's important to consider the total carbs in any food instead of just the amount of sugar. Ideally, carbs should come from whole, unprocessed foods like whole grains.

Fiber

Fiber is the part of food that is either not digested, or is only partially digested. It is crucial in a healthy diet, especially for your digestive system. Foods rich in fiber also help reduce the absorption of simple carbs (that tend to come from sugar and sweeteners).

% Daily Value (%DV)

This shows how a food fits into a 2,000 calorie/day diet. According to your current physical health and weight, you may require more or fewer calories than 2,000. In fact, if you're an adult woman who's only moderately active or not active at all, then your recommended daily calorie intake could be as low as 1,600 – 1,800. This means the values given on food labels aren't accurate for you. For this reason, always be cautious about the daily percentage values.

Ingredients

Here you see all the ingredients used in the food listed in descending order by weight. So the ingredient present in the largest amount is at the top, while the ingredient present in the smallest amount will be at the bottom. While a quick look at the top three or four ingredients may help you decide whether a particular food is good, remember that sugar and other undesirable ingredients may be disguised under several different names.

Label Claims and Their Real Meanings

Label claims can be tricky at times, especially when they are littered with words like "free", "reduced", or "low". Let's find out the truth behind these marketing buzzwords. What the label claims and what it actually means can be different:

Sugar-free = less than 0.5g of sugar

No added sugar = no sugar was added during processing…but it might naturally contain sugar

Reduced sugar = at least 25% less sugar than normal

Calorie free = 5 calories or less

Low calorie = 40 calories or less

Light = 33% fewer calories or 50% less fat

Ingredients:

Broccoli – 1 cup florets

Cucumber- 1

Celery – 1 stalk

Ginger - 1/2 thumb

Parsley – 1 handful

Green apple – 1

Lime – 1/2

Directions:

Simply process all the ingredients in your juicer and enjoy.

Nutritional Facts per Serve:

Calories: 97

Carbs: 23.5 g

Fat: 0.4 g

Protein: 1.8 g

Sugars: 18.7 g

Substitute Guide

Let's be realistic – some of your favorite recipes use refined table sugar. So, what can you use instead? Fortunately, there are many ways to convert those sugar-filled recipes to naturally sweetened ones.

For example, in many recipes, you'll find that you can simply replace one cup of refined white table sugar with approximately:

1 cup mashed ripe banana
1 cup of raisins or other sweet dried fruit
1 cup date puree (blend 3/4 cup of dried dates with 1/4 cup water)
3/4 – 1 cup of raw honey
2/3 cup of maple syrup
1 teaspoon of liquid stevia
1 teaspoon of powdered stevia

There are a few little caveats you need to be aware of:

1. Natural ingredients have variable amounts of sugar. For example, how sweet a banana is depends on the type, ripeness, growing season, and all manner of other factors.

2. Personal tastes and preferences vary. Some people like their foods sweeter than others.

3. Unlike refined table sugar, most natural sweeteners have a distinctive taste. This usually results in a tastier finished product, but it is a good idea to be mindful of the extra flavors that you're adding.

4. Most cake, loaf, muffin, and cookie recipes are pretty forgiving and you can replace the sugar with no problems at all. There are some recipes, however, which are more difficult. Things like traditional meringue rely on the chemical properties of refined white sugar. There are ways around this (for example, see Danielle Walker's recipes on her blog AgainstAllGrain.com), but it's a good idea to start with simpler recipes while you're learning how to replace refined table sugar.

5. Replacing solid white sugar with a liquid sweetener like honey will increase the amount of liquid in your recipe, so you have to counter this effect. You should decrease liquids by 1/4. For example, if the original recipe calls for 1 cup of milk, use 3/4 cup instead.

Coconut Banana Bread
Makes one loaf

Ingredients:

3 very ripe bananas, mashed

3 eggs

2 tablespoons raw honey

5 tablespoons coconut oil

1 cup coconut flour

1/2 teaspoon sea salt

2 teaspoons baking soda

1 teaspoon vanilla extract

1 teaspoon ground cinnamon

<u>*Special Diets:*</u>

If you're vegan, use 2/3 cup ground flax instead of the eggs, and add water as needed to form a sticky paste. You can replace the honey with maple syrup or any other sweetener of choice (see the substitute guide on day 18 for more ideas).

Directions:

1. Preheat the oven to 350°F (175°C).

2. Put the bananas, eggs, vanilla extract, honey, and coconut oil in a food processor and pulse until smooth. Alternatively, you can mix together by hand in a work bowl.

3. Combine all the dry ingredients together in a separate work bowl.

4. Mix the combined dry ingredients into the combined wet ingredients to form a batter.

5. Pour the batter into a greased loaf pan and place it into the oven. Bake for about an hour, or until a toothpick inserted into the center comes out clean.

Nutrition Facts per Serve:

Calories: 134

Carbs: 12.7 g

Fat: 7.1 g

Protein: 2.8 g

Sugars: 7.2 g

Day 19

How to Eat Out

You're not always going to be in the comfort of your own home where you can easily control what you're consuming. Eating out can be tricky, but there are some tips and tricks to help you watch your sugar intake.

Do Your Research

It's a good idea to spend a little time online scouting the restaurants in your local area so that you can get an idea of which ones have healthy sugar-free options. If you buy lunch on a regular basis, it's also advisable to find a couple of good, reliable options close by so that you can establish good habits and avoid simply going with whatever everyone else in the office is eating. When you're stressed and busy, you're also less likely to carefully think about what you're eating, so avoid this trap by choosing some good lunch options ahead of time.

Choose the Cuisine Carefully

Some cuisines tend to use more sugar than others, and this can often be hidden. For example, a delicious Thai curry filled with fresh vegies and lean protein is probably hiding a fair amount of palm sugar in the curry paste. This is where you need to know your own boundaries; are you willing to eat palm sugar or not? Remember that palm sugar is less refined than white table sugar, so it is healthier...but not outright healthy. This book aims to provide the information you need to make your own personal choices about what's right for you, so it's your call.

Malaysian food also often contains sugar and even sushi rolls are made from rice that has sugar added to it. In general, be cautious of sweet chili sauces, sweet and sour, honey sauces, as well as satay sauces and Chinese plum, oyster, or other sauces, all of which tend to have refined sugar added to them.

Italian food rarely has added sugar, but there are a lot of refined carbohydrates, so you need to make your own choice about this. Mexican food can be a great choice for eating out when you're sugar-free. Spanish and Greek cuisine can be good options as well.

Beware of Sauces

We already covered this a little above but be aware that sauces often contain refined sugar even if they don't taste overly sweet. This is because the combination of salty and sweet ingredients can throw your taste buds. Things like BBQ ribs are a big culprit, along with many other meat marinades, especially the sticky ones. Even a healthy salad might be slathered in a dressing packed with sugar. The safest bet is to go with simple dressings such as vinaigrettes. When in doubt, you can always just ask for olive oil and a slice of lemon and add it yourself.

Keep it Simple

Stick with simple foods like lean proteins, vegetables, beans, whole grains and nuts. If you can see the whole ingredients, you know what you're eating.

Avoid white breads and battered or crumbed food. Also be aware that some styles of baked goods – such as bagels – use sugar and other sweeteners. If you buy sandwiches for lunch, make sure you choose whole wheat and also consider flatbreads and wraps as a healthy option.

Chat with the Waiter and Chef

It's very easy to choose a healthy sounding dish and then get something completely different from what you expected. In my experience, it's far better to avoid this situation by being clear at the start. Have a chat with the waiter and be really clear about what you can and can't eat. Some wait staff have more experience with food allergies and preferences than others so, if in doubt, ask them to check with the chef. In my experience, professional chefs are always more than happy to help customers with special dietary needs. Of course, this can be especially true in natural, organic, vegetarian, gluten-free, and other specialty restaurants, health food stores, cafes and similar, as they often tend to be especially knowledgeable about ingredients and be extra willing to help you out.

Be Careful with Dessert

It goes without saying that dessert time can be particularly dangerous! If you're tempted to finish your meal with a treat, you might like to consider a fresh fruit salad. For something more satisfying, a cheese platter can be a good option for those of you who eat dairy.

Coffee or Tea?

You might have to avoid any little complementary candy or treats served with your coffee or tea, both at restaurants and cafes. I usually either give them straight to anyone else at the table who eats sugar, or give them back to the waiter immediately; if they're not in front of me, I won't eat them.

Sometimes I find going out with friends for coffee to be challenging. This is because many cafes have gorgeous cake displays and it starts to get incredibly tempting. In this situation, I often order a natural smoothie, because I know that will leave me much more satisfied and it'll be easier to resist desserts. Something like a banana and strawberry smoothie works wonders, just make sure you're clear that only whole foods are going into it, no syrups, ice-cream or similar. Also make sure any soy and nut milk is sugar-free.

Traveling

A couple of final notes for when you're traveling. Remember that you can order special meals on flights, so you might like to ask for a diabetic meal. This is also an essential time to make sure you have your own healthy snacks with you, especially in the event that a flight or any other form of transport gets delayed or cancelled! If you're travelling overseas, it's a good idea to look up the word for "sugar" in your phrase book and learn how to say "without sugar" or "no sugar". That way you can at least be sure basics like juice, coffee, and tea will be sugar-free.

Baked Figs with Honey and Rosemary
Serves 4

Why not wow friends and family at home with these easy yet delicious baked figs?

Ingredients:
Fresh figs – 8
Honey – 2 tablespoons (or use maple syrup)
Ground cinnamon – 1 teaspoon
Rosemary – 1 fresh sprig

Optional: Handful fresh ricotta

Directions:
1. Preheat your oven to 400°F (200°C).

2. Remove the tough stem from the top of each fig. Slice each fig as if you were going to cut them into quarters, but do not cut right through. Instead, only cut 2/3 of the way down. Your fig should be intact but gently open at the top.

3. Place each fig onto a baking sheet and lightly drizzle honey into the center. Sprinkle with a touch of cinnamon and a few rosemary leaves.

4. Bake for around 15 minutes, or until the figs start to caramelize. Serve as is, or crumble over a little ricotta cheese.

Nutrition Facts per Serve:
Calories: 129
Carbs: 32.5 g
Fat: 0 g
Protein: 1 g
Sugars: 28.5 g

Day 20

Alcohol

Yesterday we dealt with how to eat out, but we also need to talk about the issue of alcohol. Even though it's best to avoid drinking on this 21-Day Sugar Detox, once it's over some of you will probably want to go back to enjoying a social drink. Those of you who follow a strict Paleo diet, or anyone else who chooses not to drink, can skip over this section and go straight to today's yummy recipe. Everyone else, let's talk alcohol.

We know that alcoholic drinks are made by fermenting grains, fruits, or vegetables and that the process relies on the sugar in these ingredients. So why don't we think about the sugar in alcoholic drinks when we're trying to quit sugar?

Obviously not all drinks are created equal, so if you're looking to quit sugar but still like to enjoy the occasional drink, you should go with low-sugar options, including:

1. Dry wines (red are best)
2. Low carb beers
3. Spirits (providing they're not mixed with sugary drinks)

Make sure you avoid sweet wines, especially sweet white wines, as well as dessert wines, and ports. Liqueurs are another no-no. Champagne also contains quite a lot of sugar.

Spirits like vodka, gin, and whisky are best enjoyed neat on the rocks or with club soda. It goes without saying that you shouldn't mix them with sodas, but also be aware that tonic water is a type of soda, even though it fools you by not tasting as sweet. Fruit juice is a dangerous mixer because most bars and restaurants use highly processed "fruit drinks" which have a lot of refined sugar. If they happen to squeeze fresh juice to order, you may also consider this as a mixer.

If you are diabetic, pre-diabetic, or have any other health condition, make sure you consult your physician about your alcohol intake as even low-sugar drinks can affect your blood glucose levels.

Apart from the sugar content and health impacts of drinking, it's also well worth remembering that alcohol consists of empty calories. This means it's extremely easy to put on weight from drinking because you don't feel satisfied from the calories you're consuming. For example, each beer has around 100 calories, so even having two beers after work means you've consumed the same number of calories as a candy bar.

But let's face it; it's hard to go out with friends and see everyone drinking and sit there with nothing. In these situations, I often go for club soda with slices of fresh fruit. Most bars and restaurants have a good selection of fresh fruits on hand for cocktails, and they'll happily put some in your club soda. That way it looks like I'm drinking some kind of cocktail, so I don't need to explain my dietary choices to everyone under the sun, but I'm really only drinking water with a little fruit for interest. Better still, I'll wake up the next day feeling great!

Citrus Burst Slushy

Ingredients:
Orange – 1
Mandarin – 1
Ruby grapefruit – 1/2
Ice – 1/2 cup

Directions:
Peel the citrus, then process the ingredients in a food processor and enjoy your refreshing fruit slushy.

Nutrition Facts per Serve:
Calories: 194
Carbs: 38.2 g
Fat: 3.1 g
Protein: 5.7 g
Sugars: 14.3 g

Day 21

Final Strategies to Stay on Track

This is our last day on the 21-Day Sugar Detox so there are a couple final strategies I'd like to share with you. In a nutshell, they involve knowing your own personal weaknesses and developing strategies to cope with them.

Recognize Those Cravings

Whenever I crave something sweet, I always ask myself "what benefits does this food have?" I'm really challenging myself to see if I'm craving sugar with empty calories, or if the food is actually nutritious. If all I can think of is the pleasure of eating it, I know I'm dealing with sugar addiction! This question helps me make an informed, intelligent decision. For example, if I'm craving chocolate mousse and I know I have a recipe that's packed with fiber, potassium, vitamin K, and vitamin B6, then it's very easy to say "no" to unhealthy conventional chocolate mousse.

Prepare for Weak Moments

My biggest danger time is when I'm out running a thousand errands, accidentally skip a meal, and get really hungry. Or when I get stuck in traffic on the way home and am exhausted. Suddenly buying a chocolate bar or sugary drink seems like an easy fix. Because I know this is a weak moment, I prepare for it. I literally never leave the house without some kind of healthy snack in my purse. For me, the easiest snack is a little pack of raw nuts such as cashews and Brazil nuts, but I know other people who like to keep some whole wheat crackers with them. The snack you choose depends on your other dietary requirements, but I suggest something that keeps well so you don't need to remember it every day, and you can just leave it in your bag for a week or more.

The important thing is to recognize your week moments and put strategies in place to deal with them.

Chocolate Mousse
Makes 4 small serves or 2 generous ones

Ingredients:
Avocado – 1 large or 2 small
Raw cocoa powder – 3 tablespoons
Raw honey – 4 tablespoons (or maple syrup)
Almond milk – 1/3 cup

Directions:
Blend all the ingredients in your food processor until smooth and lusciously creamy.

Nutritional Facts per Serve:
(based on the recipe providing 4 serves)
Calories: 147
Carbs: 23 g
Fat: 6.7 g
Protein: 2 g
Sugars: 17 g

Conclusion

First of all, we've got to talk about the amazing fact that you've just successfully gone 21 days without refined table sugar – well done! I'm sure you had some moments when it wasn't easy, but you did it. Remember that it takes 3 weeks to get past the withdrawal symptoms, so you're now safely through the worst of it. Together with the wealth of information in this book – not to mention the delicious recipes – you're now well prepared to continue on your sugar-free journey.

After all, you deserve to live life to the fullest – not suffer from a myriad of health problems caused by being addicted to unhealthy refined sugar. I'm honored to have been a part of this major life change and I wish you all the health, happiness, and abundance possible in your life!

Can I Ask You a Favor?

I'm so glad you enjoyed this book enough to make it all the way to the end and I hope you've found it really useful. If you liked the book, would you be open to leaving an honest review? That would really help out other people who are looking for a book on the topic and it also helps us as a small, independent publisher.

You can leave a review by going to the relevant Amazon page in your country for this book.

Thank you!

CPSIA information can be obtained at www.ICGtesting.com
Printed in the USA
LVOW06s2223160514

386211LV00009B/174/P